CW00546382

The Definitive Alkaline Cookbook for Busy People

Make Delicious and Fast Fish Meals to Enjoy Your Diet and Lose Weight

Annalise Conley

contained within this document, including, but not limited to, —
errors, omissions, or inaccuracies.

Table of contents

Cajun Catfish

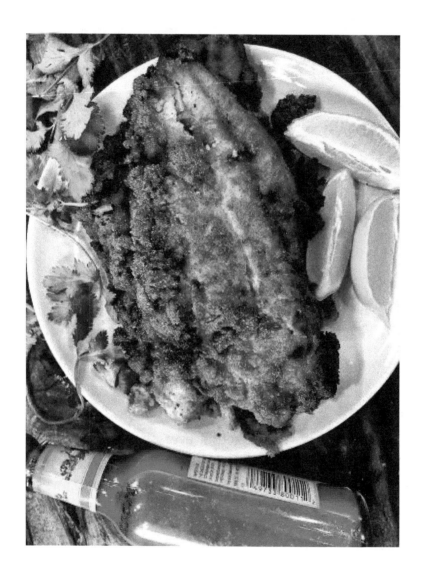

Preparation Time: 5 minutes

Cooking Time: 15 minutes

Servings: 4

Ingredients :

• 4 (8 oz.) catfish fillets

• What you'll need from store cupboard:

• 2 tbsp. olive oil

• 2 tsp. garlic salt

• 2 tsp. thyme

• 2 tsp. paprika

• 1/2 tsp. cayenne pepper

• 1/2 tsp. red hot sauce

• ¼ tsp. black pepper

• Nonstick cooking spray

Directions:

1. Heat oven to 450 degrees. Spray a 9x13-inch baking dish with cooking spray.

2. In a small bowl whisk together everything but catfish. Brush both sides of fillets, using all the spice mix.

3. Bake 10-13 minutes or until fish flakes easily with a fork. Serve.

Nutrition:

Calories 366

Total Carbs 0g

Protein 35g

Fat 24g

Sugar og

Fiber og

Cajun Flounder & Tomatoes

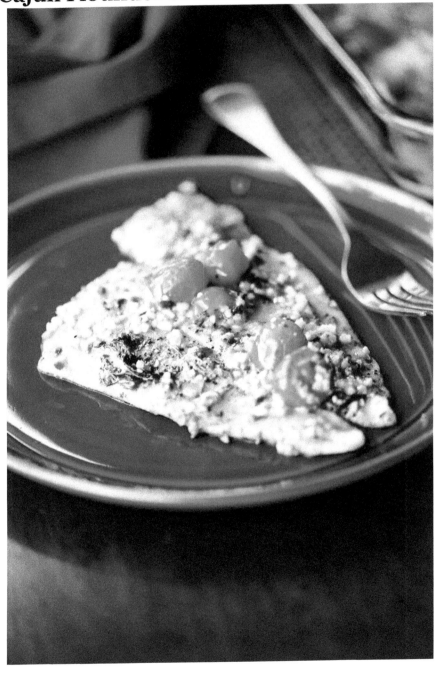

Preparation Time: 10 minutes

Cooking Time: 15 minutes

Servings: 4

Ingredients :

• 4 flounder fillets

• 2 1/2 cups tomatoes, diced

• ¾ cup onion, diced

• ¾ cup green bell pepper, diced

• What you'll need from store cupboard:

• 2 cloves garlic, diced fine

• 1 tbsp. Cajun seasoning

• 1 tsp. olive oil

Directions:

1. Heat oil in a large skillet over med-high heat. Add onion and garlic and cook 2 minutes, or until soft. Add tomatoes, peppers and spices, and cook 2-3 minutes until tomatoes soften.

2. Lay fish over top. Cover, reduce heat to medium and cook, 5-8 minutes, or until fish flakes easily with a fork. Transfer fish to serving plates and top with sauce.

Nutrition:

Calories 194

Total Carbs 8g

Net Carbs 6g

Protein 32g

Fat 3g

Sugar 5g

Fiber 2g

Cajun Shrimp & Roasted Vegetables

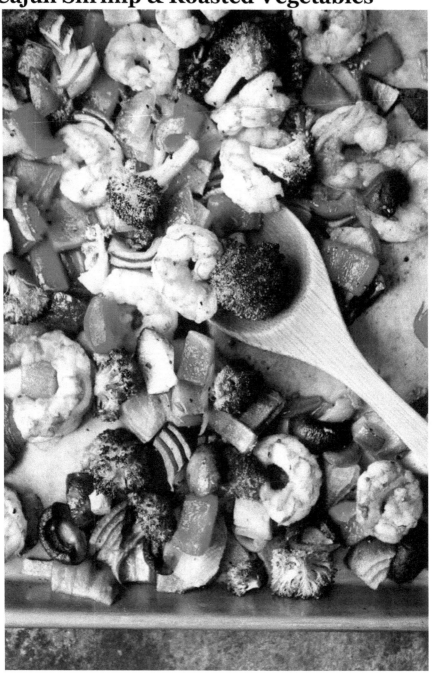

Preparation Time: 5 minutes

Cooking Time: 15 minutes

Servings: 4

Ingredients :

• 1 lb. large shrimp, peeled and deveined

• 2 zucchinis, sliced

• 2 yellow squash, sliced

• 1/2 bunch asparagus, cut into thirds

• 2 red bell pepper, cut into chunks

• What you'll need from store cupboard:

• 2 tbsp. olive oil

• 2 tbsp. Cajun Seasoning

• Salt & pepper, to taste

Directions:

1. Heat oven to 400 degrees.

2. Combine shrimp and vegetables in a large bowl. Add oil and seasoning and toss to coat.

3. Spread evenly in a large baking sheet and bake 15-20 minutes, or until vegetables are tender. Serve.

Nutrition:

Calories 251

Total Carbs 13g

Net Carbs 9g

Protein 30g

Fat 9g

Sugar 6g

Fiber 4g

Cilantro Lime Grilled Shrimp

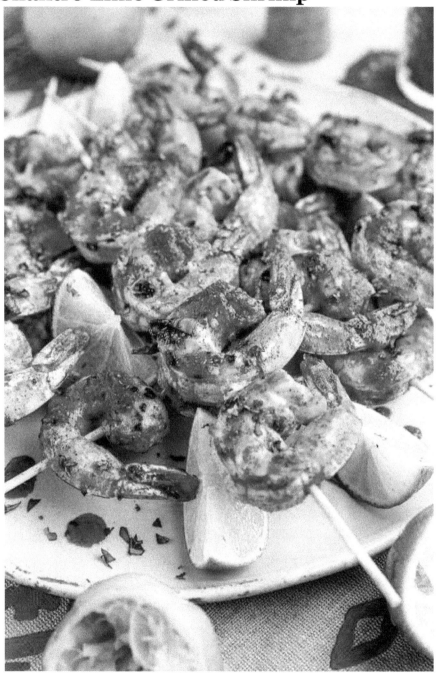

Preparation Time: 5 minutes,

Cooking Time: 5 minutes,

Servings: 6

Ingredients :

• 1 1/2 lbs. large shrimp raw, peeled, deveined with tails on

• Juice and zest of 1 lime

• 2 tbsp. fresh cilantro chopped

• What you'll need from store cupboard:

• ¼ cup olive oil

• 2 cloves garlic, diced fine

• 1 tsp. smoked paprika

• ¼ tsp. cumin

• 1/2 teaspoon salt

• ¼ tsp. cayenne pepper

Directions:

1. Place the shrimp in a large Ziploc bag.

2. Mix remaining Ingredients in a small bowl and pour over shrimp. Let marinate 20-30 minutes.

3. Heat up the grill. Skewer the shrimp and cook 2-3 minutes, per side, just until they turn pick. Be careful not to overcook them. Serve garnished with cilantro.

Nutrition:

Calories 317

Total Carbs 4g

Protein 39g

Fat 15g

Sugar 0g

Fiber 0g

Crab Frittata

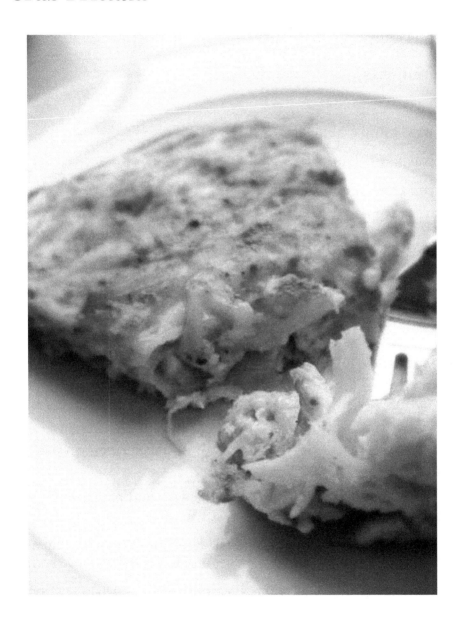

Preparation Time: 10 minutes

Cooking Time: 30 minutes

Servings: 4

Ingredients :

• 4 eggs

• 2 cups lump crabmeat

• 1 cup half-n-half

• 1 cup green onions, diced

• What you'll need from store cupboard:

• 1 cup reduced fat parmesan cheese, grated

• 1 tsp. salt

• 1 tsp. pepper

• 1 tsp. smoked paprika

• 1 tsp. Italian seasoning

• Nonstick cooking spray

Directions:

1. Heat oven to 350 degrees. Spray an 8-inch springform pan, or pie plate with cooking spray.

2. In a large bowl, whisk together the eggs and half-n-half. Add seasonings and parmesan cheese, stir to mix.

3. Stir in the onions and crab meat. Pour into prepared pan and bake 35-40 minutes, or eggs are set and top is lightly browned.

4. Let cool 10 minutes, then slice and serve warm or at room temperature.

Nutrition:

Calories 276

Total Carbs 5g

Net Carbs 4g

Protein 25g

Fat 17g

Sugar 1g

Fiber 1g

Crunchy Lemon Shrimp

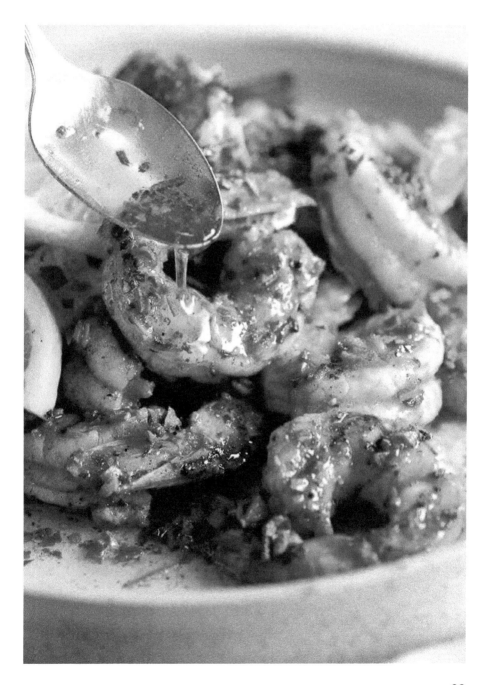

Preparation Time: 5 minutes

Cooking Time: 10 minutes,

Servings: 4

Ingredients :

• 1 lb. raw shrimp, peeled and deveined

• 2 tbsp. Italian parsley, roughly chopped

• 2 tbsp. lemon juice, divided

• What you'll need from store cupboard:

• **Servings:** cup panko bread crumbs

• 21/2 tbsp. olive oil, divided

• Salt and pepper, to taste

Directions:

1. Heat oven to 400 degrees.

2. Place the shrimp evenly in a baking dish and sprinkle with salt and pepper. Drizzle on 1 tablespoon lemon juice and 1 tablespoon of olive oil. Set aside.

3. In a medium bowl, combine parsley, remaining lemon juice, bread crumbs, remaining olive oil, and ¼ tsp. each of salt and pepper. Layer the panko mixture evenly on top of the shrimp.

4. Bake 8-10 minutes or until shrimp are cooked through and the panko is golden brown.

Nutrition:

Calories 283

Total Carbs 15g

Net Carbs 14g

Protein 28g

Fat 12g

Sugar 1g

Fiber 1g

Grilled Tuna Steaks

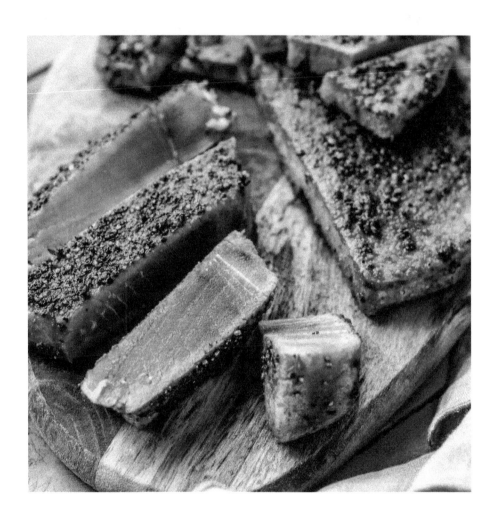

Preparation Time: 5 minutes

Cooking Time: 10 minutes,

Servings: 6

Ingredients :

• 6 6 oz. tuna steaks

• 3 tbsp. fresh basil, diced

• What you'll need from store cupboard:

• 4 1/2 tsp. olive oil

• ¾ tsp. salt

• ¼ tsp. pepper

• Nonstick cooking spray

Directions:

1. Heat grill to medium heat. Spray rack with cooking spray.

2. Drizzle both sides of the tuna with oil. Sprinkle with basil, salt and pepper.

3. Place on grill and cook 5 minutes per side, tuna should be slightly pink in the center. Serve.

Nutrition:

Calories 343

Total Carbs 0g

Protein 51g

Fat 14g

Sugar 0g

Fiber 0g

Red Clam Sauce & Pasta

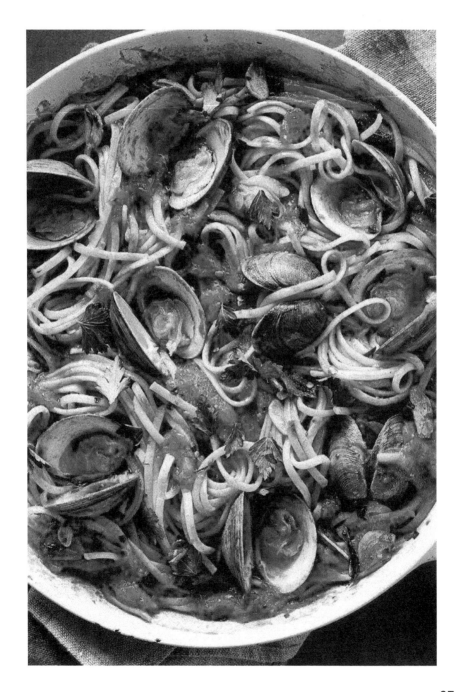

Preparation Time: 10 minutes,

Cooking Time: 30 minutes,

Servings: 4

Ingredients :

• 1 onion, diced

• ¼ cup fresh parsley, diced

• What you'll need from store cupboard:

• 2 6 1/2 oz. cans clams, chopped, undrained

• 14 1/2 oz. tomatoes, diced, undrained

• 6 oz. tomato paste

• 2 cloves garlic, diced

• 1 bay leaf

• 1 tbsp. sunflower oil

• 1 tsp. Splenda

• 1 tsp. basil

• 1/2 tsp. thyme

• 1/2 Homemade Pasta, cook & drain

Directions:

1. Heat oil in a small skillet over med-high heat. Add onion and cook until tender, add garlic and cook 1 minute more. Transfer to crock pot.

2. Add remaining Ingredients, except pasta, cover and cook for 30 minutes.

3. Discard bay leaf and serve over cooked pasta.

Nutrition:

Calories 223

Total Carbs 32g

Net Carbs 27g

Protein 12g

Fat 6g

Sugar 15g

Fiber 5g

Salmon Milano

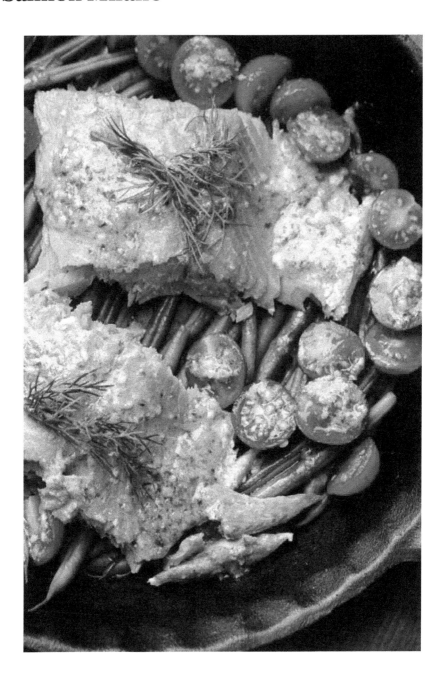

Preparation Time: 10 minutes,

Cooking Time: 20 minutes,

Servings: 6

Ingredients :

- 2 1/2 lb. salmon filet

- 2 tomatoes, sliced

- 1/2 cup margarine

- What you'll need from store cupboard:

- 1/2 cup basil pesto

Directions:

1. Heat the oven to 400 degrees. Line a 9x15-inch baking sheet with foil, making sure it covers the sides. Place another large piece of foil onto the baking sheet and place the salmon filet on top of it.

2. Place the pesto and margarine in blender or food processor and pulse until smooth. Spread evenly over salmon. Place tomato slices on top.

3. Wrap the foil around the salmon, tenting around the top to prevent foil from touching the salmon as much as possible. Bake 15-25 minutes, or salmon flakes easily with a fork. Serve.

Nutrition:

Calories 444

Total Carbs 2g

Protein 55g

Fat 24g

Sugar 1g

Fiber og

Shrimp & Artichoke Skillet

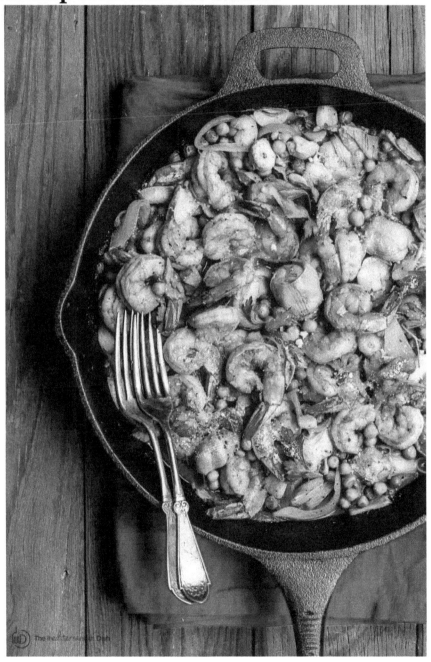

Preparation Time: 5 minutes

Cooking Time: 10 minutes

Servings: 4

Ingredients :

- 1 1/2 cups shrimp, peel & devein

- 2 shallots, diced

- 1 tbsp. margarine

- What you'll need from store cupboard

- 2 12 oz. jars artichoke hearts, drain & rinse

- 2 cups white wine

- 2 cloves garlic, diced fine

Directions:

1. Melt margarine in a large skillet over med-high heat. Add shallot and garlic and cook until they start to brown, stirring frequently.

2. Add artichokes and cook 5 minutes. Reduce heat and add wine. Cook 3 minutes, stirring occasionally.

3. Add the shrimp and cook just until they turn pink. Serve.

Nutrition:

Calories 487

Total Carbs 26g

Net Carbs 17g

Protein 64g

Fat 5g

Sugar 3g

Fiber 9g

Tuna Carbonara

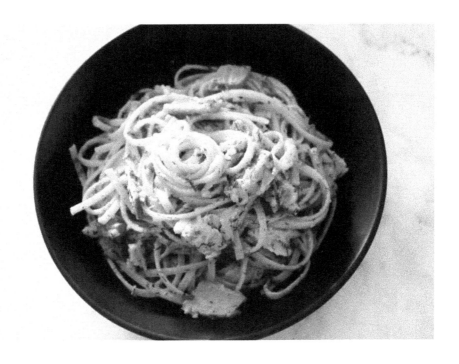

Preparation Time: 5 minutes

Cooking Time: 25 minutes

Servings: 4

Ingredients :

- 1/2 lb. tuna fillet, cut in pieces

- 2 eggs

- 4 tbsp. fresh parsley, diced

- What you'll need from store cupboard:

- 1/2 Homemade Pasta, cook & drain,

- 1/2 cup reduced fat parmesan cheese

- 2 cloves garlic, peeled

- 2 tbsp. extra virgin olive oil

- Salt & pepper, to taste

Directions:

1. In a small bowl, beat the eggs, parmesan and a dash of pepper.

2. Heat the oil in a large skillet over med-high heat. Add garlic and cook until browned. Add the tuna and cook 2-3 minutes, or until tuna is almost cooked through. Discard the garlic.

3. Add the pasta and reduce heat. Stir in egg mixture and cook, stirring constantly, 2 minutes. If the sauce is too thick, thin with water, a little bit at a time, until it has a creamy texture.

4. Salt and pepper to taste and serve garnished with parsley.

Nutrition:

Calories 409

Total Carbs 7g

Net Carbs 6g

Protein 25g

Fat 30g

Sugar 3g

Fiber 1g

Mediterranean Fish Fillets

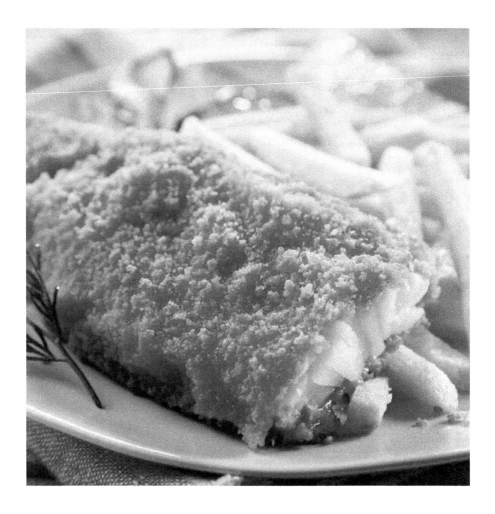

Preparation Time: 10 minutes

Cooking Time: 3 minutes

Servings: 4

Ingredients :

• 4 cod fillets

• 1 lb. grape tomatoes, halved

• 1 cup olives, pitted and sliced

• 2 tbsp. capers

• 1 tsp. dried thyme

• 2 tbsp. olive oil

• 1 tsp. garlic, minced

• Pepper

• Salt

Directions:

1. Pour 1 cup water into the instant pot then place steamer rack in the pot.

2. Spray heat-safe baking dish with cooking spray.

3. Add half grape tomatoes into the dish and season with pepper and salt.

4. Arrange fish fillets on top of cherry tomatoes. Drizzle with oil and season with garlic, thyme, capers, pepper, and salt.

5. Spread olives and remaining grape tomatoes on top of fish fillets.

6. Place dish on top of steamer rack in the pot.

7. Seal pot with a lid and select manual and cook on high for 3 minutes.

8. Once done, release pressure using quick release. Remove lid.

9. Serve and enjoy.

Nutrition:

Calories 212

Fat 11.9 g

Carbohydrates 7.1 g

Sugar 3 g

Protein 22.4 g

Cholesterol 55 mg

Creamy Avocado Cilantro Lime Dressing Recipe

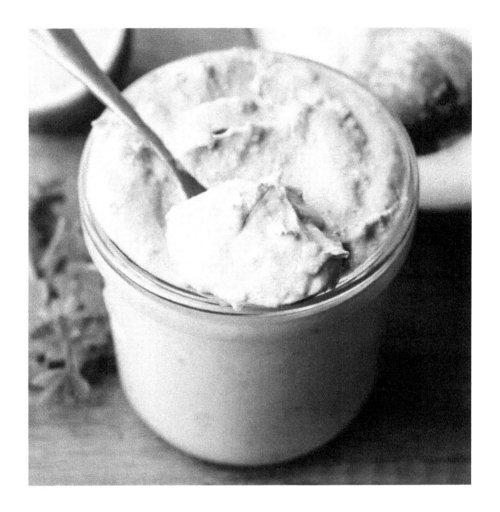

Preparation Time: 20 minutes

Cooking Time: 10 minutes

Servings: 6-8

Ingredients :

- ¼ cup olive oil
- ¼ teaspoon sea salt
- ½ cup cilantro, chopped
- ¼ cup plain goat yogurt
- Juice of ½ lime
- 1 teaspoon lime zest
- 1 avocado
- 1 clove garlic, peeled
- ½ jalapeno, chopped
- ¼ teaspoon pepper
- ½ teaspoon cumin

Directions:

1. Place/put all the Ingredients in a food processor or mixer and mix until well balanced.

Nutrition:

123 calories

1-gram protein

12 grams fat

3.6 grams carbohydrate

0.8 grams sugar

Creamy Avocado Dressing

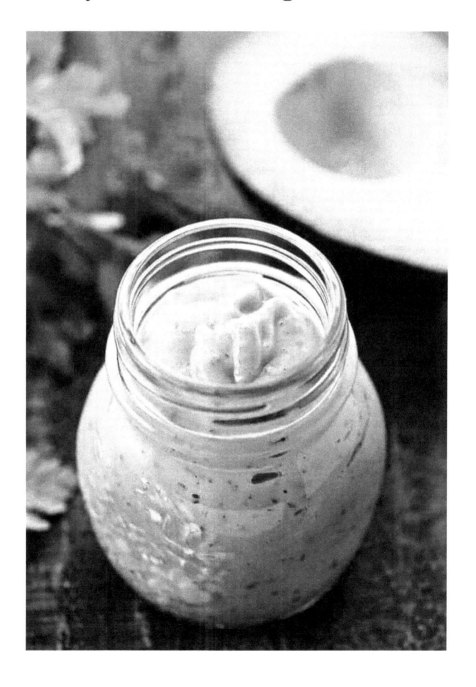

Preparation Time: 5 min

Cooking Time: 5 min

Servings: 4

Ingredients :

- 1/4 teaspoon ground black pepper
- Water, as needed
- 1 whole large avocado
- 1 clove garlic, peeled
- 1/2 tbspoon fresh lime or lemon juice
- 3 tablespoons olive oil or avocado oil
- 1/4 teaspoon kosher salt

Directions:

1. Put the peeled clove of garlic, lime or lemon juice, avocado, olive oil, salt and pepper into a mini food processor.

2. Process till smooth, stopping a few times to scrape the sides down. Thin the salad dressing out with some water (1/4 cup to 1/2 cup) before a perfect consistency is achieved.

3. Maintain/keep at least a week in an airtight container, but 3 to 4 days is best.

Nutrition:

Calories: 38.2

Total fat: 2.6 grams

Saturated fat: 0.6 grams

Cholesterol: 1.2 milligrams

Sodium: 8.8 milligrams

Potassium: 76.9 milligrams

Total carbohydrate: 3.6 grams

Dietary fiber: 1.0 grams

Sugars: 0.9 grams

Southwestern Avocado Salad Dressing

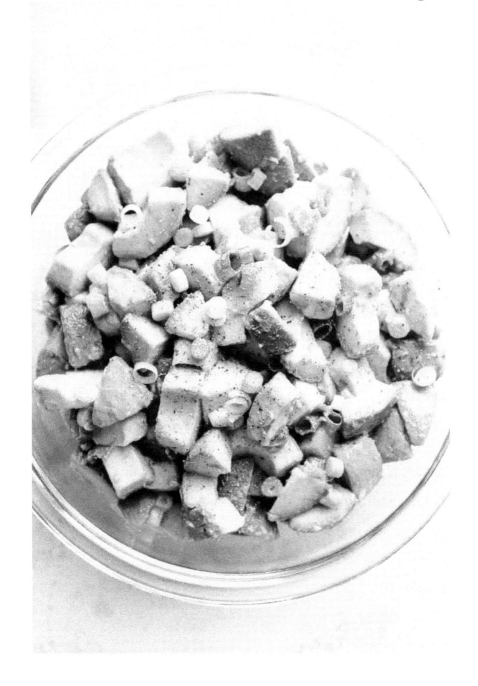

This avocado salad dressing salad packs a punch of cilantro and lime flavor. It is full of good avocado fat and adds a delicious twist to every salad in the southwest!

Preparation Time: 5 minutes

Cooking Time: 30 minutes

Servings: 8

Ingredients :

• 1 ripe avocado

• 1 cup buttermilk

• 1/2 teaspoon garlic powder

• 1/2 teaspoon chipotle chili powder

• 1/2 teaspoon salt

• 1/4 cup cilantro

• Juice of 1/2 lime

• 1 teaspoon ranch seasoning powder homemade or store bought

Directions:

1. Break the avocado in half, extract the pit from the flesh and scoop the skin.

2. Attach all the other Ingredients together to a mixer.

3. Blend in until creamy and smooth.

4. Prior to serving, refrigerate for 30 minutes.

5. Keeps in the refrigerator for 3 days.

Nutrition:

Calories: 61

Calories from fat: 36

Total fat: 4 grams

Saturated fat: 1 gram

Cholesterol: 3 milligrams

Sodium: 237 milligrams

Potassium: 162 milligrams

Total carbohydrates: 4 grams

Dietary fiber: 1 gram

Sugars: 1 gram

Protein: 1 gram

Lemon Avocado Salad Dressing

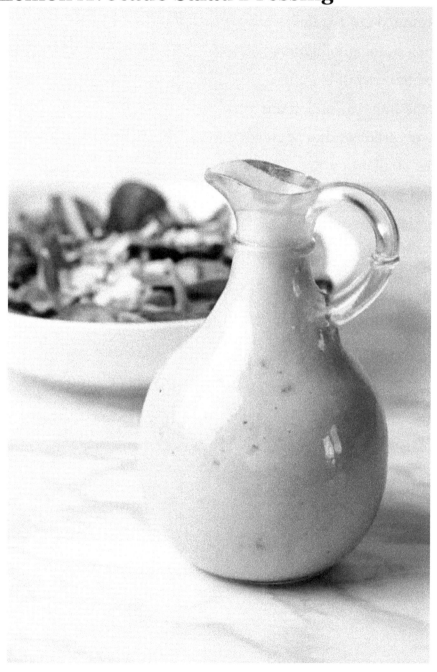

This creamy dressing, with its strong lemon taste, is a refreshing change of pace, not one that you can find on the shelves of the groceries. My uncle shared the recipe with me in california.

Preparation Time: 5 minutes

Cooking Time: 5 minutes

Servings: 2-3

Ingredients :

• 2 tablespoons olive oil

• 1 garlic clove, minced

• 1/2 teaspoon seasoned salt

• 1 medium ripe avocado, peeled and mashed

• 1/4 cup water

• 2 tablespoons sour cream

• 2 tablespoons lemon juice

• 1 tbspoon minced fresh dill or 1 teaspoon dill weed

• 1/2 teaspoon honey

• Salad greens, cherry tomatoes, sliced cucumbers and sweet red and yellow pepper strips

Directions:

1. In a blender, combine the first nine Ingredients; cover and process until blended. Serve with salad greens, tomatoes, cucumbers and peppers. Store in the refrigerator.

Nutrition:

Calories: 38.2

Total fat: 2.6 grams

Saturated fat: 0.6 grams

Cholesterol: 1.2 milligrams

Sodium: 8.8 milligrams

Potassium: 76.9 milligrams

Total carbohydrate: 3.6 grams

Dietary fiber: 1.0 grams

Sugars: 0.9 grams

Protein: 0.8 grams

Avocado Salad With Bell Pepper And Tomatoes

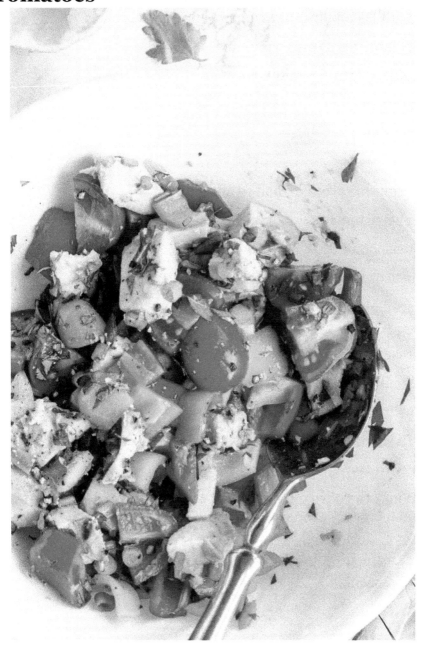

Avocado shells make convenient vessels made with the scooped-out flesh for a vivid salad. The dressing is flavored with lime juice, garlic and a pinch of cayenne. The salad may also be used as a quesadillas topping, or as a new filling for tacos.

Preparation Time: 5 minutes

Cooking Time: 5 minutes

Servings: 2-3

Ingredients :

• Coarse salt

• 1 firm, ripe avocado, halved and pitted

• 6 cherry tomatoes, halved

• 1 teaspoon extra-virgin olive oil

• Juice of 1/2 lime

• 1 scallion, trimmed and thinly sliced

• 1 tbspoon chopped fresh cilantro leaves, with whole leaves for garnish

• 1 small garlic clove, minced

• Pinch of cayenne pepper

• 1/2 yellow bell pepper, ribs & seeds removed, diced

Directions:

1. Whisk the olive oil, lime juice, garlic, and cayenne together in a small bowl. Season with the salt.

2. From the avocado halves, scoop out flesh, conserve shells and chop. Switch to a bowl and add chopped cilantro, bell pepper, onions, scallion.

3. Drizzle with salt and season with dressing. Stir gently to mix. Mix spoon into allocated containers. Garnish with whole leaves of cilantro and serve right away.

Nutrition:

Calories: 424

Fiber: 16.36 grams

Saturated fat: 5 grams

Carbohydrates: 31.25 grams

Fat: 34.63 grams

Protein: 6.6 grams

Avocado Egg Salad

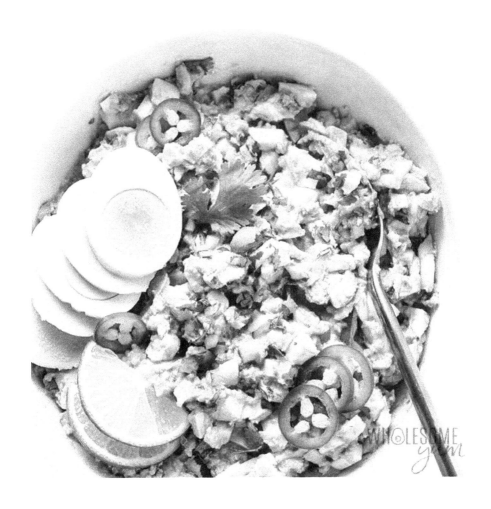

Preparation Time: 10 minutes

Cooking Time: 5 minutes

Servings: 4

Ingredients :

- 2 eggs, hard boiled
- 1 avocado, finely chopped
- 3 tablespoons boiled corn
- 1 tomato, thinly chopped
- 1 tablespoon extra-virgin olive oil
- Salt to taste
- 1 tablespoon lemon juice
- 3 green onions, chopped

Directions:

1. In a large bowl, whisk in chopped avocado and lemon juice.

2. In the same bowl, mix it with other Ingredients, except for tomato.

3. Serve on slices of bread with sliced tomatoes.

Nutrition:

Calories: 119

Fat: 8.7 grams

Cholesterol: 125 milligrams

Carbohydrates: 3.4 grams

Protein: 7.2 grams

Avocado Caprese Salad

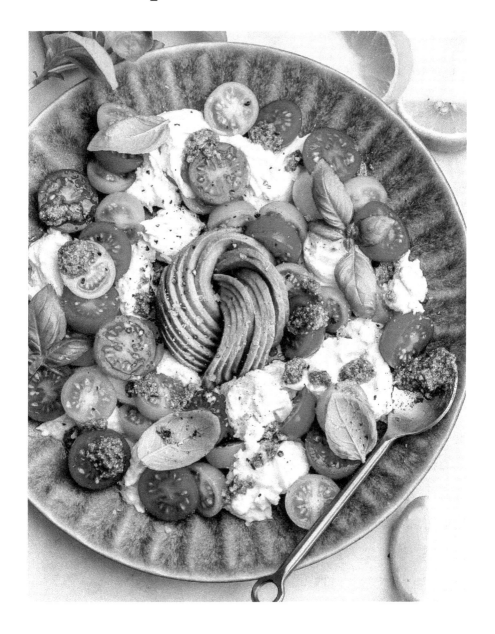

Preparation Time: 5 minutes

Cooking Time: 5 minutes

Servings: 1

Ingredients :

- 1 1/2 teaspoons balsamic vinegar
- Generous pinch of sugar/dollop of honey
- 3 slices fresh mozzarella cheese
- Fresh basil leaves
- 2 cups fresh arugula
- 2-3 campari or cocktail style tomatoes sliced
- 1/2 avocado pitted and sliced
- 1 tablespoon extra-virgin olive oil
- Kosher salt and freshly ground black pepper

Directions:

1. In a serving bowl, add the arugula, onion, avocado slices, and mozzarella. Fill with leaves of broken or slivered basil. With the balsamic vinegar, sugar or honey, whisk the extra virgin olive oil in a small bowl and season with kosher salt and freshly ground black pepper to taste and pour over the salad. Throw coat and serve.

Nutrition:

Calories: 164.2

Fat: 11.8 grams

Cholesterol: 10.0 milligrams

Carbohydrates: 11.6 grams

Fiber: 4.7 grams

Sugar: 5 grams

Protein: 5.4 grams

Avocado Salmon Salad With Arugula

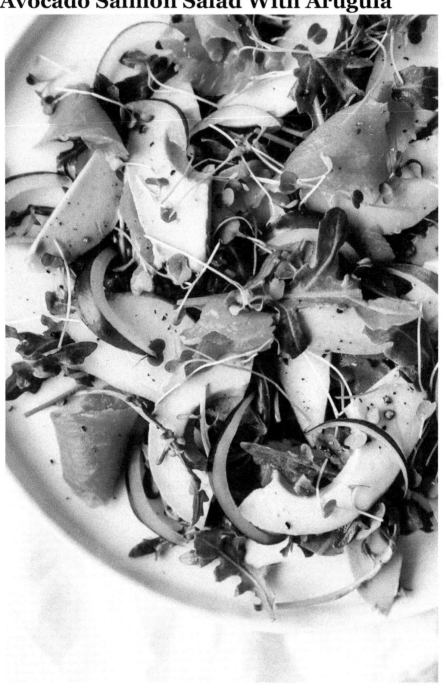

Preparation Time: 10 minutes

Cooking Time: 5 minutes

Servings: 1

Ingredients :

• 2 green onions, sliced thinly

• 8 cherry tomatoes, halved (or a mix of yellow and red)

• ¾ pound salmon fillet

• 1 avocado, pitted, peeled and chopped

• 1 small (raw) zucchini, thinly sliced in half moons

• 4 radishes, thinly sliced

• 1 recipe avocado citrus dressing

Directions:

1. Preheat to 400 ° f on oven. Line a small saucepan with parchment paper.

2. Arrange salmon on the pan, skin down, and bake for 10 to 12 minutes until just cooked.

3. Warm slightly, cut fat, flake flesh and set aside.

4. Divide arugula between serving plates. Top with salmon and avocado, courgettes, red onion and tomatoes.

5. Serve in citrus dressing with creamy avocado

Nutrition:

Calories: 320

Fat: 32 grams

Cholesterol: 5 milligrams

Potassium: 210 milligrams

Carbohydrates: 6 grams

Fiber: 3 grams

Protein: 6 grams

Wild Rice And Black Lentils Bowl

Preparation Time: 10 minutes

Cooking Time: 40 minutes

Servings: 4

Ingredients :

• Wild rice

• 2 cups wild rice, uncooked

• 4 cups spring water

• ½ teaspoon salt

• 2 bay leaves

• Black lentils

• 2 cups black lentils, cooked

• 1 ¾ cups coconut milk, unsweetened

• 2 cups vegetable stock

• 1 teaspoon dried thyme

• 1 teaspoon dried paprika

• ½ of medium purple onion; peeled, sliced

• 1 tablespoon minced garlic

• 2 teaspoons creole seasoning

• 1 tablespoon coconut oil

• Plantains

• 3 large plantains, chopped into ¼-inch-thick pieces

• 3 tablespoons coconut oil

• Brussels sprouts

- 10 large brussels sprouts, quartered

- 2 tablespoons spring water

- 1 teaspoon sea salt

- ½ teaspoon ground black pepper

Directions:

1. Prepare the rice: take a medium pot, place it over medium-high heat, pour in water, and add bay leaves and salt.

2. Bring the water to a boil, then switch heat to medium, add rice, and then cook for 30–40 minutes or more until tender.

3. When done, discard the bay leaves from rice, drain if any water remains in the pot, remove it from heat, and fluff by using a fork. Set aside until needed.

4. While the rice boils, prepare lentils: take a large pot, place it over medium-high heat and when hot, add onion and cook for 5 minutes or until translucent.

5. Stir garlic into the onion, cook for 2 minutes until fragrant and golden, then add remaining Ingredients for the lentils and stir until mixed.

6. Bring the lentils to a boil, then switch heat to medium and simmer the lentils for 20 minutes until tender, covering the pot with a lid.

7. When done, remove the pot from heat and set aside until needed.

8. While rice and lentils simmer, prepare the plantains: chop them into ¼-inch-thick pieces.

9. Take a large skillet pan, place it over medium heat, add coconut oil and when it melts, add half of the plantain pieces and cook for 7–10 minutes per side or more until golden-brown.

10. When done, transfer browned plantains to a plate lined with paper towels and repeat with the remaining plantain pieces; set aside until needed.

11. Prepare the sprouts: return the skillet pan over medium heat, add more oil if needed, and then add brussels sprouts.

12. Toss the sprouts until coated with oil, and then let them cook for 3–4 minutes per side until brown.

13. Drizzle water over sprouts, cover the pan with the lid, and then cook for 3–5 minutes until steamed.

14. Season the sprouts with salt and black pepper, toss until mixed, and transfer sprouts to a plate.

15. Assemble the bowl: divide rice evenly among four bowls and then top with lentils, plantain pieces, and sprouts.

16. Serve immediately.

Nutrition:

Calories: 333

Carbohydrates: 49.2 grams

Fat: 10.7 grams

Protein: 6.2 grams

Lemony Salmon

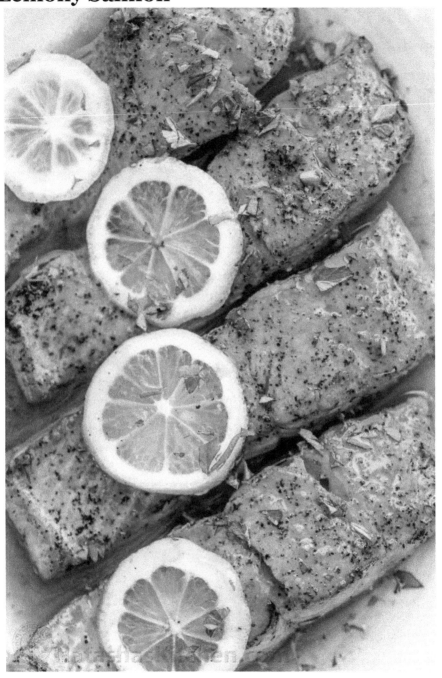

Preparation Time: 10 minutes

Cooking Time: 3 Minutes

Servings: 3

Ingredients :

• 1 pound salmon fillet, cut into 3 pieces

• 3 teaspoons fresh dill, chopped

• 5 tablespoons fresh lemon juice, divided

• Salt and ground black pepper, as required

Directions:

1. Arrange a steamer trivet in Instant Pot and pour ¼ cup of lemon juice.

2. Season the salmon with salt and black pepper evenly.

3. Place the salmon pieces on top of trivet, skin side down and drizzle with remaining lemon juice.

4. Now, sprinkle the salmon pieces with dill evenly.

5. Close the lid and place the pressure valve to "Seal" position.

6. Press "Steam" and use the default time of 3 minutes.

7. Press "Cancel" and allow a "Natural" release.

8. Open the lid and serve hot.

Nutrition:

Calories: 20

Fats: 9.6g,

Carbs: 1.1g,

Sugar: 0.5g,

Proteins: 29.7g,

Sodium: 74mg

Shrimp With Green Beans

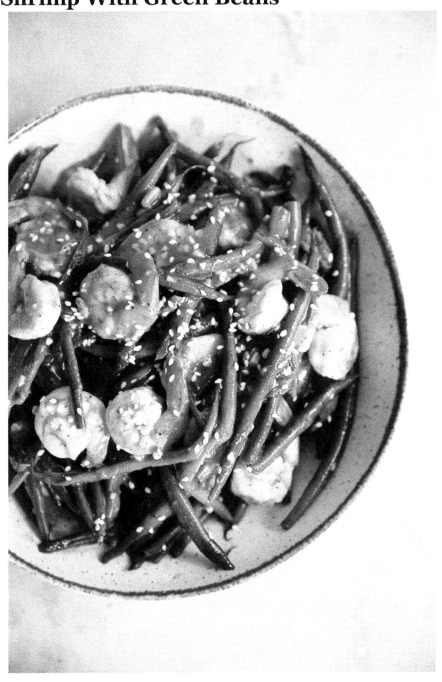

Preparation Time: 10 minutes

Cooking Time: 2 Minutes

Servings: 4

Ingredients :

- ¾ pound fresh green beans, trimmed
- 1 pound medium frozen shrimp, peeled and deveined
- 2 tablespoons fresh lemon juice
- 2 tablespoons olive oil
- Salt and ground black pepper, as required

Directions:

1. Arrange a steamer trivet in the Instant Pot and pour cup of water.

2. Arrange the green beans on top of trivet in a single layer and top with shrimp.

3. Drizzle with oil and lemon juice.

4. Sprinkle with salt and black pepper.

5. Close the lid and place the pressure valve to "Seal" position.

6. Press "Steam" and just use the default time of 2 minutes.

7. Press "Cancel" and allow a "Natural" release.

8. Open the lid and serve.

Nutrition:

Calories: 223,

Fats: 1g,

Carbs: 7.9g,

Sugar: 1.4g,

Proteins: 27.4g,

Sodium: 322mg

Crab Curry

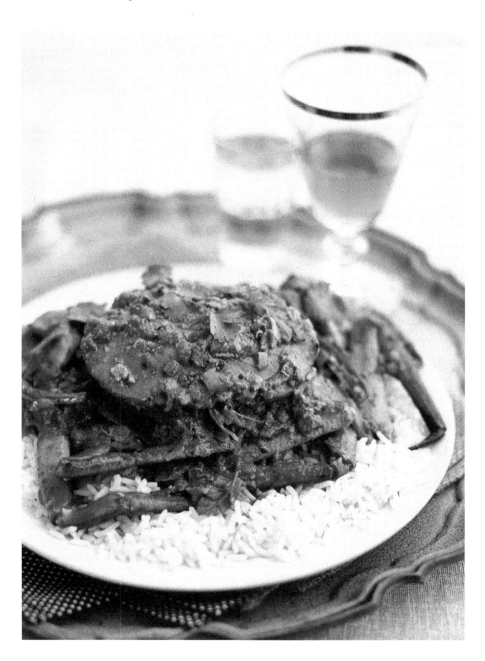

Preparation Time: 10 minutes

Cooking Time: 20 Minutes

Servings: 2

Ingredients :

• 0.5lb chopped crab

• 1 thinly sliced red onion

• 0.5 cup chopped tomato

• 3tbsp curry paste

• 1tbsp oil or ghee

Directions:

1. Set the Instant Pot to sauté and add the onion, oil, and curry paste.

2. When the onion is soft, add the remaining **Ingredients** and seal.

3. Cook on Stew for 20 minutes.

4. Release the pressure naturally.

Nutrition:

Calories: 2;

Carbs: 11;

Sugar: 4;

Fat: 10;

Protein: 24;

GL: 9

Mixed Chowder

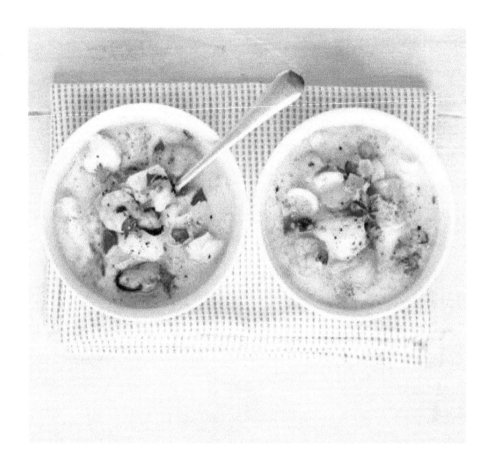

Preparation Time: 10 minutes

Cooking Time: 35 Minutes

Servings: 2

Ingredients :

- 1 lb fish stew mix

- 2 cups white sauce

- 3 tbsp old bay seasoning

Directions:

1. Mix all the Ingredients in your Instant Pot.

2. Cook on Stew for 35 minutes.

3. Release the pressure naturally.

Nutrition:

Calories: 320;

Carbs: 9;

Sugar: 2;

Fat: 16;

Protein: GL: 4

Mussels In Tomato Sauce

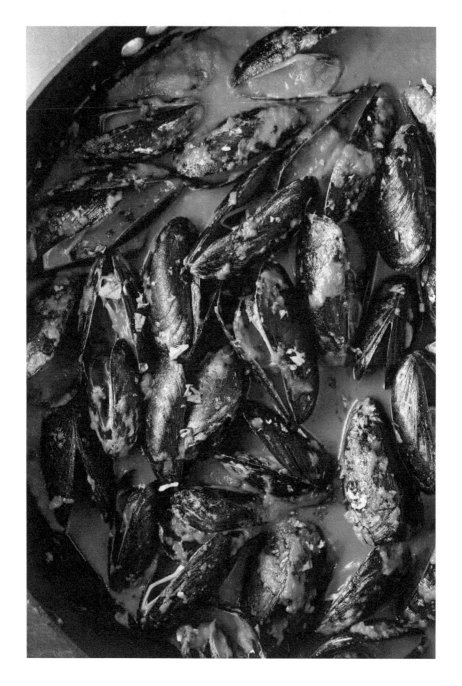

Preparation Time: 10 minutes

Cooking Time: 3 Minutes

Servings: 4

Ingredients :

• 2 tomatoes, seeded and chopped finely

• 2 pounds mussels, scrubbed and de-bearded

• 1 cup low-sodium chicken broth

• 1 tablespoon fresh lemon juice

• 2 garlic cloves, minced

Directions:

1. In the pot of Instant Pot, place tomatoes, garlic, wine and bay leaf and stir to combine.

2. Arrange the mussels on top.

3. Close the lid and place the pressure valve to "Seal" position.

4. Press "Manual" and cook under "High Pressure" for about 3 minutes.

5. Press "Cancel" and carefully allow a "Quick" release.

6. Open the lid and serve hot.

Nutrition:

Calories: 213,

Fats: 25.2g,

Carbs: 11g,

Sugar: 1

Proteins: 28.2g,

Sodium: 670mg

Citrus Salmon

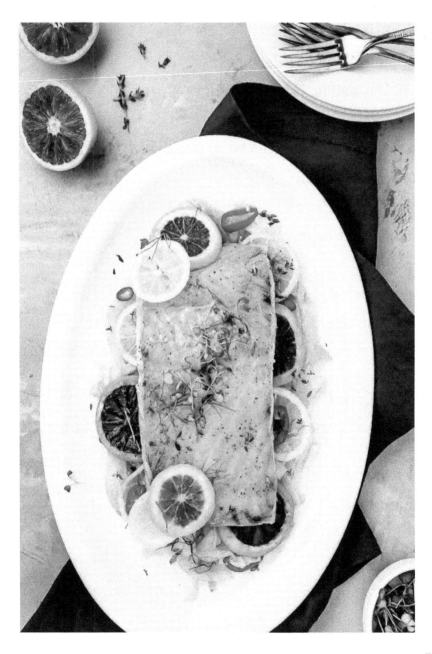

Preparation Time: 10 minutes

Cooking Time: 7 Minutes

Servings: 4

Ingredients :

• 4 (4-ounce) salmon fillets

• 1 cup low-sodium chicken broth

• 1 teaspoon fresh ginger, minced

• 2 teaspoons fresh orange zest, grated finely

• 3 tablespoons fresh orange juice

• 1 tablespoon olive oil

• Ground black pepper, as required

Directions:

1. In Instant Pot, add all Ingredients and mix.

2. Close the lid and place the pressure valve to "Seal" position.

3. Press "Manual" and cook under "High Pressure" for about 7 minutes.

4. Press "Cancel" and allow a "Natural" release.

5. Open the lid and serve the salmon fillets with the topping of cooking sauce.

Nutrition:

Calories: 190,

Fats: 10.5g,

Carbs: 1.8g,

Sugar: 1g,

Proteins: 22

Sodium: 68mg

Herbed Salmon

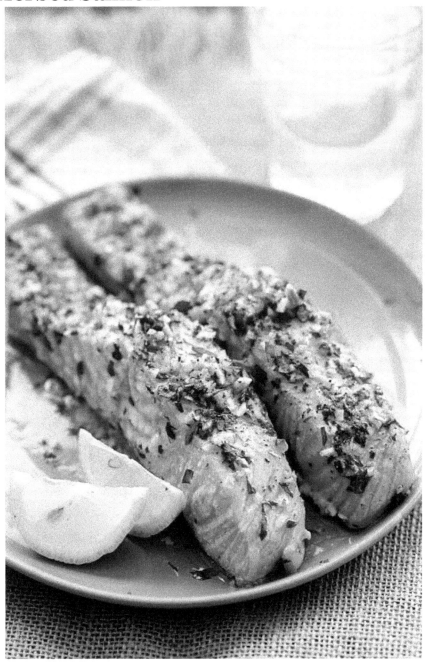

Preparation Time: 10 minutes

Cooking Time: 3 Minutes

Servings: 4

Ingredients :

• 4 (4-ounce) salmon fillets

• ¼ cup olive oil

• 2 tablespoons fresh lemon juice

• 1 garlic clove, minced

• ¼ teaspoon dried oregano

• Salt and ground black pepper, as required

• 4 fresh rosemary sprigs

• 4 lemon slices

Directions:

1. For dressing: in a large bowl, add oil, lemon juice, garlic, oregano, salt and black pepper and beat until well co combined.

2. Arrange a steamer trivet in the Instant Pot and pour 11/2 cups of water in Instant Pot.

3. Place the salmon fillets on top of trivet in a single layer and top with dressing.

4. Arrange 1 rosemary sprig and 1 lemon slice over each fillet.

5. Close the lid and place the pressure valve to "Seal" position.

6. Press "Steam" and just use the default time of 3 minutes.

7. Press "Cancel" and carefully allow a "Quick" release.

8. Open the lid and serve hot.

Nutrition:

Calories: 262,

Fats: 17g,

Carbs: 0.7g,

Sugar: 0.2g,

Proteins: 22.1g,

Sodium: 91mg

Salmon In Green Sauce

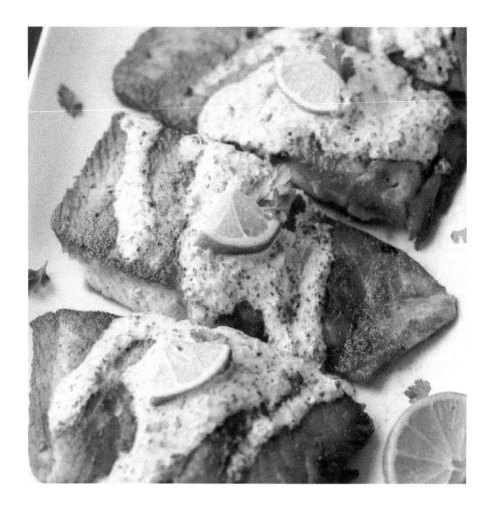

Preparation Time: 10 minutes

Cooking Time: 12 Minutes

Servings: 4

Ingredients :

• 4 (6-ounce) salmon fillets

• 1 avocado, peeled, pitted and chopped

• 1/2 cup fresh basil, chopped

• 3 garlic cloves, chopped

• 1 tablespoon fresh lemon zest, grated finely

Directions:

1. Grease a large piece of foil.

2. In a large bowl, add all Ingredients except salmon and water and with a fork, mash completely.

3. Place fillets in the center of foil and top with avocado mixture evenly.

4. Fold the foil around fillets to seal them.

5. Arrange a steamer trivet in the Instant Pot and pour 1/2 cup of water.

6. Place the foil packet on top of trivet.

7. Close the lid and place the pressure valve to "Seal" position.

8. Press "Manual" and cook under "High Pressure" for about minutes.

9. Meanwhile, preheat the oven to broiler.

10. Press "Cancel" and allow a "Natural" release.

11. Open the lid and transfer the salmon fillets onto a broiler pan.

12. Broil for about 3-4 minutes.

13. Serve warm.

Nutrition:

Calories: 333,

Fats: 20.3g,

Carbs: 5.5g,

Sugar: 0.4g,

Proteins: 34.2g,

Sodium: 79mg

Braised Shrimp

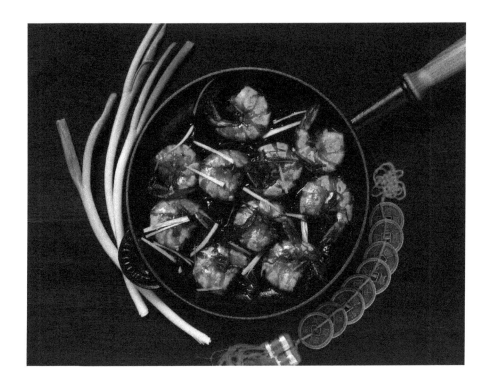

Preparation Time: 10 minutes

Cooking Time: 4 Minutes

Servings: 4

Ingredients :

• 1 pound frozen large shrimp, peeled and deveined

• 2 shallots, chopped

• ¾ cup low-sodium chicken broth

• 2 tablespoons fresh lemon juice

• 2 tablespoons olive oil

• 1 tablespoon garlic, crushed

• Ground black pepper, as required

Directions:

1. In the Instant Pot, place oil and press "Sauté". Now add the shallots and cook for about 2 minutes.

2. Add the garlic and cook for about 1 minute.

3. Press "Cancel" and stir in the shrimp, broth, lemon juice and black pepper.

4. Close the lid and place the pressure valve to "Seal" position.

5. Press "Manual" and cook under "High Pressure" for about 1 minute.

6. Press "Cancel" and carefully allow a "Quick" release.

7. Open the lid and serve hot.

Nutrition:

Calories: 209,

Fats: 9g,

Carbs: 4.3g,

Sugar: 0.2g,

Proteins: 26.6g,

Sodium: 293mg

Shrimp Coconut Curry

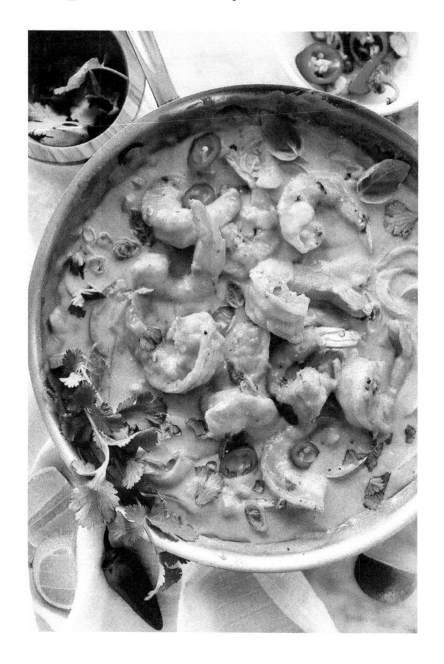

Preparation Time: 10 minutes

Cooking Time: 20 Minutes

Servings: 2

Ingredients :

- 0.5lb cooked shrimp
- 1 thinly sliced onion
- 1 cup coconut yogurt
- 3tbsp curry paste
- 1tbsp oil or ghee

Directions:

1. Set the Instant Pot to sauté and add the onion, oil, and curry paste.

2. When the onion is soft, add the remaining Ingredients and seal.

3. Cook on Stew for 20 minutes.

4. Release the pressure naturally.

Nutrition:

Calories: 380;

Carbs: 13;

Sugar: 4;

Fat: 22;

Protein: 40;

GL: 14

Trout Bake

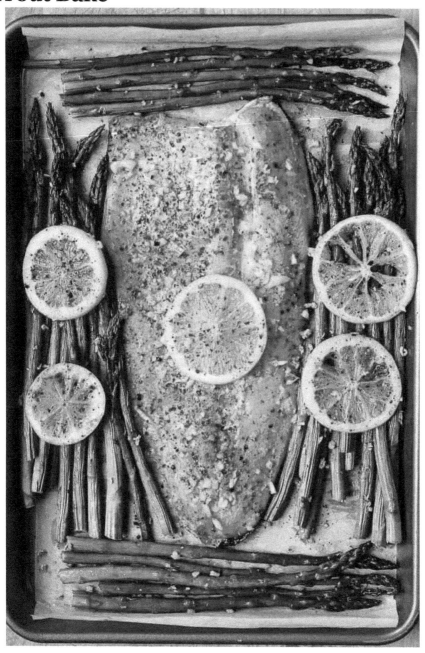

Preparation Time: 10 minutes

Cooking Time: 35 Minutes

Servings: 2

Ingredients :

- 1lb trout fillets, boneless
- 1lb chopped winter vegetables
- 1 cup low sodium fish broth
- 1tbsp mixed herbs
- sea salt as desired

Directions:

1. Mix all the Ingredients except the broth in a foil pouch.

2. Place the pouch in the steamer basket your Instant Pot.

3. Pour the broth into the Instant Pot.

4. Cook on Steam for 35 minutes.

5. Release the pressure naturally.

Nutrition:

Calories: 310;

Carbs: 14;

Sugar: 2;

Fat: 12;

Protein: 40;

GL: 5

Sardine Curry

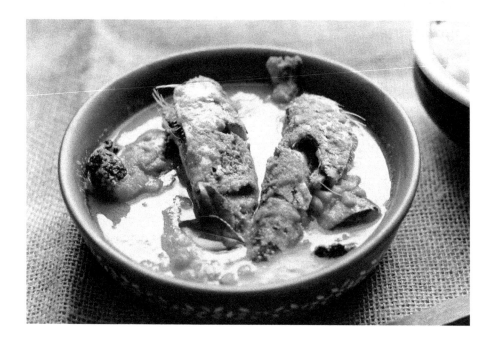

Preparation Time: 10 minutes

Cooking Time: 35 Minutes

Servings: 2

Ingredients :

• 5 tins of sardines in tomato

• 1lb chopped vegetables

• 1 cup low sodium fish broth

• 3tbsp curry paste

Directions:

1. Mix all the Ingredients in your Instant Pot.

2. Cook on Stew for 35 minutes.

3. Release the pressure naturally.

Nutrition:

Calories: 320;

Carbs: 8;

Sugar: 2;

Fat: 16;

Protein:

GL: 3

Swordfish Steak

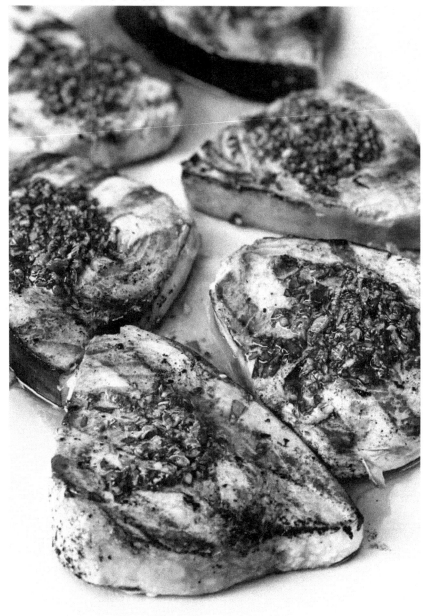

Preparation Time: 10 minutes

Cooking Time: 35 Minutes

Servings: 2

Ingredients :

- 1lb swordfish steak, whole

- 1lb chopped Mediterranean vegetables

- 1 cup low sodium fish broth

- 2tbsp soy sauce

Directions:

1. Mix all the Ingredients except the broth in a foil pouch.

2. Place the pouch in the steamer basket for your Instant Pot.

3. Pour the broth into the Instant Pot. Lower the steamer basket into the Instant Pot.

4. Cook on Steam for 35 minutes.

5. Release the pressure naturally.

Nutrition:

Calories: 270;

Carbs: 5;

Sugar: 1;

Fat: 10;

Protein: 48;

GL: 1

Lemon Sole

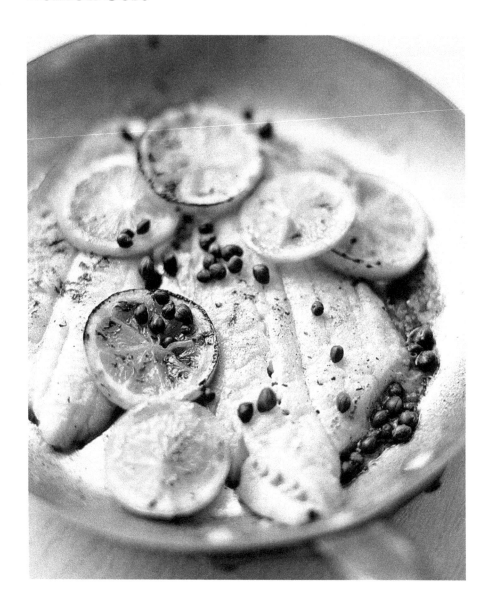

Preparation Time: 10 minutes

Cooking Time: 5 Minutes

Servings: 2

Ingredients :

- 1lb sole fillets, boned and skinned
- 1 cup low sodium fish broth
- 2 shredded sweet onions
- juice of half a lemon
- 2tbsp dried cilantro

Directions:

1. Mix all the Ingredients in your Instant Pot.

2. Cook on Stew for 5 minutes.

3. Release the pressure naturally.

Nutrition:

Calories: 230;

Carbs: Sugar: 1;

Fat: 6;

Protein: 46;

GL: 1

Tuna Sweet Corn Casserole

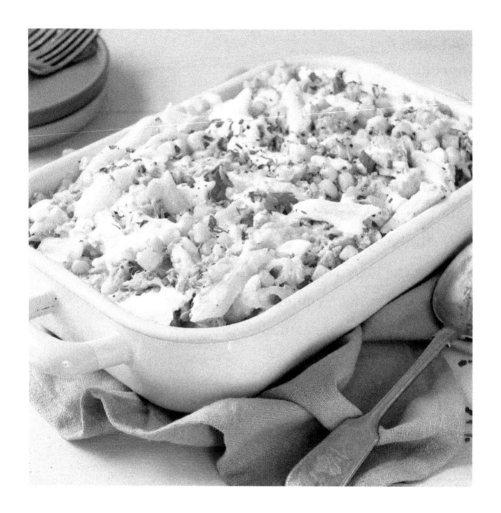

Preparation Time: 10 minutes

Cooking Time: 35 Minutes

Servings: 2

Ingredients :

- 3 small tins of tuna
- 0.5lb sweet corn kernels
- 1lb chopped vegetables
- 1 cup low sodium vegetable broth
- 2tbsp spicy seasoning

Directions:

1. Mix all the Ingredients in your Instant Pot.

2. Cook on Stew for 35 minutes.

3. Release the pressure naturally.

Nutrition:

Calories: 300;

Carbs: 6 ;

Sugar: 1 ;

Fat: 9 ;

Protein: ;

GL: 2

Lemon Pepper Salmon

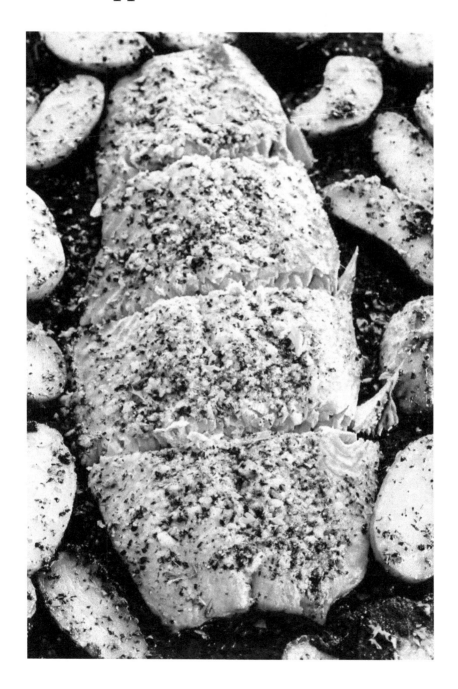

Preparation Time: 10 minutes

Cooking Time: 10 Minutes

Servings: 4

Ingredients :

- 3 tbsps. ghee or avocado oil
- 1 lb. skin-on salmon filet
- 1 julienned red bell pepper
- 1 julienned green zucchini
- 1 julienned carrot
- ¾ cup water
- A few sprigs of parsley, tarragon, dill, basil or a combination
- 1/2 sliced lemon
- 1/2 tsp. black pepper
- ¼ tsp. sea salt

Directions:

1. Add the water and the herbs into the bottom of the Instant Pot and put in a wire steamer rack making sure the handles extend upwards.

2. Place the salmon filet onto the wire rack, with the skin side facing down.

3. Drizzle the salmon with ghee, season with black pepper and salt, and top with the lemon slices.

4. Close and seal the Instant Pot, making sure the vent is turned to "Sealing".

5. Select the "Steam" setting and cook for 3 minutes.

6. While the salmon cooks, julienne the vegetables, and set aside.

7. Once done, quick release the pressure, and then press the "Keep Warm/Cancel" button.

8. Uncover and wearing oven mitts, carefully remove the steamer rack with the salmon.

9. Remove the herbs and discard them.

10. Add the vegetables to the pot and put the lid back on.

11. Select the "Sauté" function and cook for 1-2 minutes.

12. Serve the vegetables with salmon and add the remaining fat to the pot.

13. Pour a little of the sauce over the fish and vegetables if desired.

Nutrition:

Calories 296,

Carbs 8g,

Fat 15 g,

Protein 31 g,

Potassium (K) 1084 mg,

Sodium (Na) 284 mg

Baked Salmon With Garlic Parmesan Topping

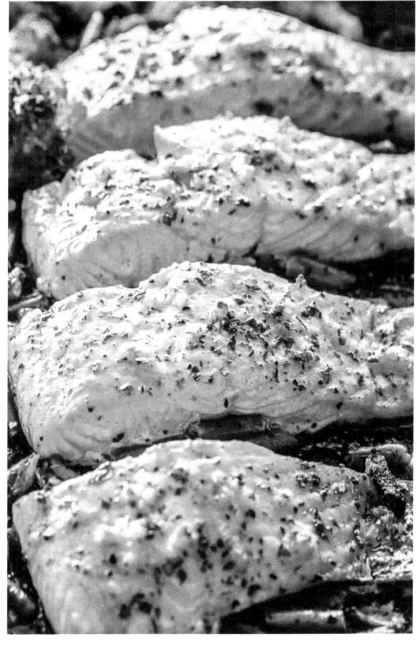

Preparation Time: 5 minutes,

Cooking Time: 20 minutes,

Servings: 4

Ingredients :

• 1 lb. wild caught salmon filets

• 2 tbsp. margarine

• What you'll need from store cupboard:

• ¼ cup reduced fat parmesan cheese, grated

• ¼ cup light mayonnaise

• 2-3 cloves garlic, diced

• 2 tbsp. parsley

• Salt and pepper

Directions:

1. Heat oven to 350 and line a baking pan with parchment paper.

2. Place salmon on pan and season with salt and pepper.

3. In a medium skillet, over medium heat, melt butter. Add garlic and cook, stirring 1 minute.

4. Reduce heat to low and add remaining Ingredients. Stir until everything is melted and combined.

5. Spread evenly over salmon and bake 15 minutes for thawed fish or 20 for frozen. Salmon is done when it flakes easily with a fork. Serve.

Nutrition:

Calories 408

Total Carbs 4g

Protein 41g

Fat 24g

Sugar 1g

Fiber 0g

Blackened Shrimp

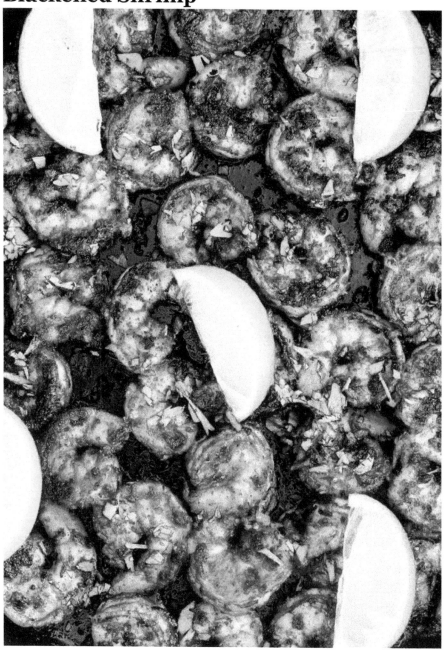

Preparation Time: 5 minutes

Cooking Time: 5 minutes

Servings: 4

Ingredients :

- 1 1/2 lbs. shrimp, peel & devein
- 4 lime wedges
- 4 tbsp. cilantro, chopped
- What you'll need from store cupboard:
- 4 cloves garlic, diced
- 1 tbsp. chili powder
- 1 tbsp. paprika
- 1 tbsp. olive oil
- 2 tsp. Splenda brown sugar
- 1 tsp. cumin
- 1 tsp. oregano
- 1 tsp. garlic powder
- 1 tsp. salt
- 1/2 tsp. pepper

Directions:

1. In a small bowl combine seasonings and Splenda brown sugar.

2. Heat oil in a skillet over med-high heat. Add shrimp, in a single layer, and cook 1-2 minutes per side.

3. Add seasonings, and cook, stirring, 30 seconds. Serve garnished with cilantro and a lime wedge.

Nutrition:

Calories 252

Total Carbs 7g

Net Carbs 6g

Protein 39g

Fat 7g

Sugar 2g

Fiber 1g

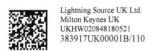

9 781802 695342